LIFE AFTER HEART BREAK OF A WOMAN

The secret way out for women

Dews & Drops

INTRODUCTION

We are in a world full of emotional pain and romantic loss for women. At this time, the incidence of divorce and break up is now beyond rampant, it's now a regular sequence that most girls and ladies must experience break up , divorce and heart breaks.   This life challenge have now spread like a wild fire to most part of the world that theres's hardly any part of the globe where

where women, a lot of them are crying and weeping every day as as they face a life of rejection and impossible dreams.

My attention got into this silent destroyer of ladies after I saw what my sisters have gone through and currently going through, with no hope of succor and I feel their pains always, and yet they don't know largely because they can not tell every one these secret things, but as a regular baller, I know these things and I can see it in the many failures they are facing, most of them cause by the heartless MEN.

I don't mean like these ladies are innocent them selves men are guilty, I mean from experience both men and women are romance vampires. But this book is a series catalogue written by a combination of writters and experts in different topics and i merely collected by consent their articules to bring different and diverse context to this work and enrich my readers. What i also mean is that just as women are suffering from deception and break up,men are also suffering severe break ups as well and many have committed or attempted suicide. So this one is for the woman and another one will be written for the men. I have suffered break up many times too, so i will also want to learn how to avoid this event like the others.

To day, if I look at my parents and their parents (my grand parents), i never see such a pain. My father and mother argue all the time and even fight , but separation was like having a cold shower in hell fire. So for me to see this now becoming a common sight is a surprice. But on a closer look, i can spot the difference.

PURPOSE OF THIS BOOK

The purpose or objective of this book, is what is on its name. This work seeks to expose some secrets to women in their quest to survive wicked men. First it will explain what we mean by heartbreak, it would then move to indicate what causes heartbreak. And it would show the women some few signals to show that heart break might be at the corner and how to prevent it. Prevention in this case may not mean stopping it, or what is the essence of an abusive relationship? The prevention could be how to work on the reasons that would be listed below, but also how to prepare for it and prevent it from being an heartbreak. Lastly, it would list some ways to move on from heart break and even thrive in it. Thanks as you read.

According to WIKIPEDIA, a Broken Heart is a metaphor for the intense emotional stress or pain one feels at experiencing great and deep longing. The concept is cross-cultural , often cited with reference to unreciprocated or lost love. The clear definition here makes reference to losing some one you think you love or you can not do without. (Note how I use it, some one you think you love. Love is like every human issue, subjective, it is subject to lies,it is subject to what ever idear good or bad that any one thinks at a point in time)

Heartbreak can be such an intense experience, that even scientists have correctly suggested that it might feel the same way if not more than a physical pain, because it is possible to die from an experience of Heartbreak!

From a personal experience, I think Heartbreak is an experience you wouldn't wish your arch enemy, not to talk of people close to you. Because heart break can even render a special person useless transforming them into a shadow till the end of his or her life. I have seen a lot of ladies who end up becoming a recluse shag and a waste, a walking shadow with no hope or ambition for the future, and in some of these cases, the men who cause these women to break down are them selves living in great abandon, some are living in opulence and don't even remember the ashes they left, which is also why we have seen horror cases were women take laws into their own hands and wreak havoc on the unsuspecting heartbreakers. Like one here the man was having another affair behind his girl friend and when she knew, the lure the man to come spend a night at her place and when the two of them have finish a night bed rumble and the happy tired man was sleeping, the venomenous woman rose up in the dark and go pick a bowl of acide she hid some where, and pured the burning substance on the sleeping man's face and he wailed from deep inside sleep and the woman pack her bags and ran away from the house. Today the man lost his two eyes as the acide virtually gleaned away his entire face, such that you don't even see eye socket and his face melted. The man is crying till date and no one knows where the woman is or even who she is as the man don't have eyes to identify her. Perhaps she might even be among the mourners in his house. The man is now , well a dead man walking.

Heart break is more of unreciprocated love and perhaps a lost love. A woman loves , or believes she loves her a man (lesbian relationship is not represented here), and only for her to feel that her man may not be totally committed to her. She may feel he is not kindle to her like she is to him.

It can even go further, for instance it can begin in unreciprocated love to lost love. The problem could start gradually till it goes into a break up.

I have witnessed a lot of these. A woman watch as her home or man is taken over by another woman and she losses out and many go into a dark place and don't recover for life.

Heartbreak in the most form in this context, is for the man to tell the woman that he is no longer interested in their union and goes away.

Heartbreak could also come in the form where the man begins to misbehave and constantly provoke the woman. When a man has another woman, he usually engages this method to break from the old flame. They will no longer attend to her needs and may be the man don't have courage to tell the woman it is over, he will just disengage gradually till they are no more in talking terms and the end.

Again some men will, like this is common to educated ones, the man would just go away without warning. Like he may say his going some where to spend a short period and say his goodbyes and in his mind that's the final good bye. And the woman will not see him again. This one is usually the most painful, since infact there would be no prior problem manifest, or altercation. This case is where the man had already brokeup with the lady in his mind and then

do it gradually. By and large breakup heartbreak is a painful situation.

Although this for a is strictly for a woman challenge, i can relate it with my

experience because the feelings are the same. In my own experience, when I

had this kind of heartbreak, there was a hook in my heart, I lost a lot. And

most times you feel you can't come out of losing some one you thought you

love. But like every thing about the human life…it's vanity and you can

actually live without any one including your parents if you can put your mind

at rest and chill out, i mean your parents are more important than any other

persons, so one can always survive a heartbreak and even thrive and succeed.

And in the final analysis, no one not even a love one is indispensable! So a

woman that is adamant about keeping a man at all cost despite red light and

believe he belong to her alone, is perhaps playing like the fool. Because the

man, and men when they move on to another woman, timing of action is

always of the essence for the woman left behind. She don't have time to

pretend like its not happening, she has to move fast and secure her self as

quickly as possible. At the onset, men always guess right that the woman they

are cutting lose won't come to her senses fast to also go in the other

direction. I mean you can cry for the love but you must not wait for the love, your life must not be in suspended animation , while the man is romancing a strange woman. If the woman can throw him away fast, it might bring peace to all parties and if the man was on a fishing expedition in troubled waters , he will quickly suffer and strain and tension may come into his new chase. A fast woman will secure one important factor, her peace of mind. If the mind is lost then emotional torture will set in and the life of such a woman will not be the same again and recovery period in this case will be long and tedious. So time to move on is of the essence.

A stich in time always saves nine. Princes Diana of England died due to her longing to keep prince Charles, while Charles had already moved on.

DIFFERENCE BETWEEN BREAKUP AND HEARTBREAK

A **<u>breakup</u>** is usually a mutual disengagement, a situation where the two parties have already grown tired of each other and wont miss each other if one or both parties leaves at the same time. In other words, in break up it is common for both parties to realise the incompartibility to accept departure. But it is also not common for the two to agree to break at the same time, some one must be the one to reach breaking point first and take action to

leave the union. But the remaining partner won't be complaining, perhaps in

most case the vector partner in crisis will be the one to leave last.

Again what should be noted is that it is also common for partners who broke

up to come back together. That may not be possible with heartbreak.

A **<u>Heartbreak</u>**, as mentioned in the introduction, is a situation where one

party is totally committed to the union, while the other party wants out. And

the party that wants out goes on to terminate the union at the detriment of

the other party. And they can come back on oly few occasions but that would

also be after they must have both gone into several numerous other

relationships and then return to the vomit, but in most cases heartbreak

couples don't return back together.

GENERAL REACTIONS TO HEARTBREAK

Loss Of Apetite: most women in a state of heartbreak experience a total

loss of apetite. They can no longer eat or even drink, they become inured to food. They can stay for hours without food and this will then take a toll on their health stability and cognitive abilities. Again this shouldn't be a surprice. Usually when you are in a very sad mood, food may no longer interest you, like wise a woman in a state of emotional distress may no longer see the appeal in food, but some can even now eat beyond healthy proportion and food may even become their solace.

Emotional breakdown : These women in this situation will not think

right no more. Their thought will be in the wind, they will be crying day and night. Some will be pained by the investment on that person and some will be probably pain that may be they can not get that type of person again. Some ladies even lose weight and become empty shells, some become like shadows wailking in the dark, I have also heard some who begin to see nignt mares and dream of the man for a long time. I have seen some who quickly go into alcohol and drugs and hemp as they could not survive without help and I have seen some who go into a rehab, I mean psychiatric hospitals and homes, and that mean many fall into insanity. Some usually can move on but they are very few in numbers. But for me all these are totally uneccessary, as no body

don't have adequate replacement.

Hatred And Suspision of Men : When a woman passes through a

heartbreak, especially if she were still very young, she would develop a

general apathy for men. Some may develop extreme hatred such that she may

no longer be interested in any more romantic lesion with a man. Many of

these type of women become lesbian or just loose interest in men generally.

Some may not exhibite their sadness in this anomie, rather they may go ahead

to look for men, but with deep sitted suspicion and animosity.

Loss of Self Esteem. Some of these women can lose their sense of self

worth, they can doubt their quality and for good reason. This is especially if

she felt for good reason that the man left her for a physically more beautiful

lady , they nearly don't recover from it and they probably totally lose hope in

getting a good man in future and if they see one , they become hunted by

what happened last time. And when a lady loses her sense of importance, she

become easy pickings for marauding serial heart breakers, which means she may now beome wortless to other men and they may have to dump her again.

Many these kind of ladies end up in brothels or become prostitutes and sluts.

Romantic failures and unmarried : Again I have noticed that some

women who go through heart breaks and especially serial losers, some may

never even find love no more. I have seen formerly beautiful models who

quickly became recluse and old shacks after suffering angonising heartbreaks. I

mean heartbreaks is a plague to be avoided due to its lasting consequences.

Some of these men dump these ladies late and as such water must have passed

the bridge, I mean these ladies may have become useless to society having

invested their lives to these male predators.

DEATH : Death they say is the end of every thing, conversely a heartbreak

could also be the end of every thing for some women, I mean I have seen

women who went on to marry after a painful heartbreak and ended up barren

in the new husband house. They just became barren and infertile suddenly

and we can attribute this to hormonal problems. The heartbreak could affect

her whole processing system.

We have seen many cases where women die, either by suicide or by depression. Many women who had their big dreams torn to shreads, may not be able to live life after the event. And this is why prevention is always better than a cure. A woman can always prevent a heartbreak by breaking her self from mental slavery. If a woman can break off by her self, she will heal more quickly than if she is dump suddenly. And this is why a woman must be able to see the symptoms and avoid it the pitfalls rather than go into the ditch.

My friend Paul Hickman will speak on the next chapter

WHAT CAUSES A MAN TO DUMP A WOMAN

by   Paul Hickman

I would have liked to write of both sides, but my moderator asked that I write on why a man will dump or leave a lady. I want my readers to understand that dumping a woman in this context, is different from some thing like DIVORCE. Please lets take note.

8 in 10 men in united states will tell you that they have dump a girl or two or even a dozen. Personally I have had to leave or end relationship with a few dozen girls since I started dating from 7th grade. Also the figure is the same in other western world and divorce is just slightly lower. In Africa, it is a bit lower to 7 in 10 men , who abandons their lady at a pont in time. Now for some men i will agree that it is like a sport and they continue to dump every lady they have just like this crazy guy, Leonardo Dicaprio, or like late Hefner, or you may wannar mention brad pitt or this Afleck and Jeniffa lopez drama.

Some of these men dump ladies like a sport, but you will also see that some popular men are still with their wives…..men like Clooney, men like will smith, men like Jay Z and Beyoncy, men Barack Obama and michelle, men like David Beckam, Men like prince William, many can remember Denzel Washington.

So some great men are still thriving with their wives , despite the noises in their family and in some we don't even hear noise.

Question, ladies might ask is why are some men still with their wives , while a lot other have dump them. Am also sorry, because I stated that divorce will not be the context here,so am sorry for these married men I mentioned, but it's the same thing and lets follow the ball.

Men dump women due to not one but various reasons. I also remember that I left each of those ladies based , in many ways, different peculiar issues. And I have also being dump by a lot of ladies too and some of them, am still scratching my head to know the reason why but, that is the human phenomenon. Any thing about human issues are always normative and subjective and totally devoid of any single definition. So likewise in human relationship, you will never know what is in the mind of people until they act them out.

Love like any other human issue can grow old, and if there was no substance in it or if both parties refuse to adjust to the partnership or if one partner is acidic and has no remedy, then the love will quicklywear out and die! This must be said, that even in situation where the two partners are doing well and there seem to be no societal challenge, love can also become old and boring and the partners will need time apart to build it back, the interest.

Due to the kind of society we now have where most activities have been lost to internet craze and automation, some relationships can quickly become boring or monotonous and uninteresting. Inmost cases this aint the fault of no particular party. You just don't see substance in a relationship any more. I have seen cases where a romance ended it sweetness or essence in just a day and I mean that a man, after just one night stand or just after one night or a day may quickly lose total interest in a lady. And the main point here is that the lady in question may not know. She may not know that her prince charming has lost interest in her, just that very day and if assuming that lady has invested her emotion or hope into that man, then what will happen is gonna be like a slow motion heartbreak!

That's that a man who has become emotionally detached in just a day or so may even pretend and stay for for years, probably exploiting the woman in other ways. And I have seen a situation where a man is collecting money from one woman to secretly use to spend on a new lady he is keeping secretly. This is common when, or if the lady is richer or she is a model or big catch.

Don't also forget that some times the man will only lose interest after a while like weeks, months or years or even after marriage! The bottom line is that when a man loses interest, it becomes a matter of when not if , he will dump the lady. And if at this stage, whether a day or more , the lady can see this and get these signals, then she can quickly divest from the man and probably end it or begin to cut away gradually too and this will ultimately limit her over all exposure to the vagaries of the man. When this happens then there wont be killer heartbreaks but probably a break up.

In most cases repeating the same activies over a period might bring fatigue and a lack of interest, even sex some times it can become boring if it becomes same thing, although its seldome. But a woman who does the same thing can make the man lose interest. Some women don't know how to spice up the relationship and they don't bother to go and learn what they can add to bring more interest.

And if married or not married some times you just get tired of see some one and this can be or this is in most cases temporal and interest returns but that depends on other events like distance and proximity or it can be a permanent fissure. But then it is also possible that the interest never dies because some souls are spiritually tied for life. So then if the two are hot on it , it will not matter the love will remain there for ever.

I remember looking at the situation in former president George Walker Bush, I mean the old late president of united states. The love between him and his wife went on till the verey end and both were nearly close in age, and aged together. Now after the wife died, like we understood that before she died she was under a drug therapy to manage an ailment and then she suddenly announced that she will stop usage of the drug due to the great inconvinence the usage is causing her and she wanted to be left alone. I was shocked that she died just few months after she made that pronouncement. Then also surprisingly, her husband also died the following year! And you will be curious about such a close bond of souls, I think we can go study that family.

KEEPING SORDID SECRETS

A man can lose interest in a lady just for the same reasons a lady or ladies lose interests in men.   The same way a lady will hate for a man to keep secrets, men are far worse at accepting secrets. They lose their minds and take irrational actions after discovery. So a lady must be very careful in keeping secrets that could destroy her home, its better she don't do it or she better let the man know or eliminate the vector

I remember a situation where a guy and a lady were so tight for some time and every thing seem pointed to a wedding, but at this time this couple had not have sex yet and yet the man was just as infatuated as the lady. But the lady didn't tell the man that she has done mexactomy or removed on breast due infection on one of her breasts. She had placed a fake breast there so there were differences. Thus when on one accassion emotion carried them and in the heat, they took off cloths and had sex and it was during this time that the man collided with this issue and he was shocked and his infatuation vanished there immediately. Don't forget that the woman haven placed a fake breast there, had thought it would be no different and she did not tell the man.

Now when the man made that discovery, he too did not ask the lady any question, he just went on an investigation secretly and that's when the girl people unwithingly told him the news. He did as if he was fine but he was making preparations to travel out and he began to look for another lady and then went to do a secret wedding and soon he disappeared with the new lady and this older lady was heartbroken! But she didn't know that the love had vanished even years ago.

Several reasons.....infact a lady can also make a relationship die even as she is desperately working to sustain it. And I cant also say if theres any particular thing a lady can do to not make her romance turn boring, this all lies on individualistic tendencies and diversity. HUMAN beings can never be satistfied

Doing shit at the back and thinking he don't know : Women always have this clever or may be stupid idea that men are dumb! Oh men don't see colors , men don't know what's going on.   Totally wrong! Men truly are not nosey dogs but they are clear eye vultures. Men may and I mean just some of them, some of men don't usually go hunting for crimes, and they take a lady on face value. If a man meets a lady that he loves, he at that time will not think she can do any wrong. When a man loves a woman, she will be as clean as an angel in his eyes for those moment, even if she is a demon or a witch, he will not know and a woman can easily deceive him.   But most times in their bumbling, and fumbling , their eyes are still very sharp and since the woman would be under the false believe that he is not focus on her and she lose her guard, then he will see or notice some thing or even read some thing from her action. And immediately a man smells a rat, he will not just investigate the presing problem, he will investigate the entire life of the woman and take action bases on that.

Now let me tell a story From a problem that is similar to what I listed above .

I had a beautiful family aunt who usually showered me with goodies when I was still a teenager, even at my young age I usually secretly crush on her, i just knew she was a model and she was truly an amazon. There was this middle age man she was dating, who drop her with his car every day I could remember, then this man travelled to another distant country to work and prepare for their marriage and union.   Truly , during this time when this man was away, from what I knew for I followed out some times, this lady was having side flings with other men in the area. I knew of one but I later heard of a lot of escapades of this lady. She was beautiful and every damn man wanted to have a slice and they paid heavily. Heard she was sending some of this money to the spouse abroad, although a don't know where she would tell him she got the money.   You have to know that this lady (Rose), would have had a concrete believe that her spouse would never know that she ever opened her thighs to any other dick! But some years went by and this spouse of hers begin to also reduce his connection, and she was at a loss but she had a total faith that her prince was engrossed with work and will soon return to fetch her. But then this prince had infact married another woman in that foreign land, and am not sure any one knows when he did that, but this aunt of mine later heard this like a fake news, but it turn out true. Am sure she would have killed the man if she got near but that was it she lost it and she was close to 41 years(the man was gone for 7 years).

She later tried to make me sleep with her but I refuse, but my regret was that I didn't even sit down to know why she took that decision, I just thought it was dirty. But as I see that she cant have a child today , I begin to wonder may be she was trying to beat menopause and I regret not helping her. She now a total recluse and poor with no job and doesn't dress good no more and when I call her, she said she don't wanner see men because she is no longer the woman she used to be. My sisters do see her by chance and they say she is just like a dirty maid now, just walking the street like an orphan!

This is what heartbreak can do to a woman, which is why a hard working , beautiful and loyal loving lady must watch out for it and escape it because its effects could be devastating and permanent. And also heart break is no respecter of beauty or breain or loyalty. Just take a look at the world model Naomi, she had all the beauty yet every man had to run , even ones she spent on. So every woman must be aware of these things.

Some ladies unintentionally begin to use slur words for their man immediately they start relationship. To them its part of the romance but for some men it's a crises for the romance. Some don't bother to do those respectful things they usually do when the man was just new to them and some men may even like it but some men will react negatively to it and think of ending the show.

So if a woman is not or doesn't really care to show some decorum to her man , then that man may think she is not a good girl to be with. There are little things a lady may do, which she don't really care about but the man will see it as insulting.

I remember a man who had this hot girl he was infatuated with and took her every where. The man was a football team coach, and his team performance begin to suffer as he was more focus on his new catch. One of the things they do was go eat at the joint some times, but as the man's life style began to generate discussion, he told his lady that he wants her to start living like a home woman now, he wants to balance his life so that he wont be kicked or sacked from his job. He meant that they wont be spending to much time on trivial . This lady, (whom I can presume was a former club girl) refused to integrate and adjust. She kept pestering the couch for out door dinners and lunch and it became nagging. The man was taking big salary from this job and

he knew he can be sacked if he don't put his acts together.   Then one

Saturday morning they were on the bed and the man was thinking about to

strategise on the team problems, then suddenly the lady tapped him, and said

she has seen a new joint that they must go today. The man went totally

beserk, but he didn't shout it out, then he camly asked her what is wrong if

she go to the kitchen and prepare some thing for them and stop talking shit!

She wasn't having that, she told him to go do it him self if that's took his bath

and dressed up and left.   This man was divorced from his wife of many years

and wanted some thing new, but here he was with no happiness but a slut

who wanted to ruin him financially he thought. When he was with his wife

he never knew a woman can hate the kitchen and he seldom go to eat at joint

and his wife don't always like to go with him and to cap it, it was during those

years that he achieved his acclaim as an astute coach . but now he cant even do

a job.   The man filed for divorce and and returned to his old wife. And this

woman cried for many years and went bankrupt , sold the car and properties

the man left and after the rent of the house was due after some years, she was

back on the street and doing the shitty job and till date she don't see no more

husband. She is now a shadow .

Hygiene means cleanliness to avoid diseases or caring for the body.

When a woman doesn't take care of her body in area of cleaning her key regions then some men may freak out and want out. There are men,like me who will try to correct and direct her where theres lack so that she will be ok, most of the men would not correct. Most men like one of my childhood friends

Once told me he thought WOMEN NEVER FART, until his former girl friend did it and he could not stand it and they quickly broke up.   I mean some men grow up to see women like these angels who don't do no wrong, who smell good all the time like their aunties. And they are totally derailed and shock when they meet a dirty woman.   So any woman who don't take care of her mouth, her cloths, her undies, her toilet usage, her bath room usage, her finger nails, her eyes, her kitchen habits, her room habits, and farts unecessarily will be courting danger of a break up of divorce. And the worse thing as I mentioned on this one is that men who hate those things would not talk, they will probably see the woman as an antequated, untrained, illiterate, or a village dweller or a slum dweller.   Any dirty girl will be seen as a slum

dweller by most men. I cant say too much on hygiene , but generally hygiene

don't usually rank high as the reason for breakup, I guess ordinarily most

women are even more clean than men. Again that may be debateable , as I

would want to feel that men in their normal slow eye may not quickly spot a

dirty woman in their house, or even her dirtiness may even be sexualy

charging. But when it get to the head, a man may run from a dirty woman

period.

HAVING OTHER CLOSE MEN OR BOY FRIENDS

Now just like men would say, women too usually may have a previous love

interest or boy friend and some women do have numerous. If a man discovers

that his girl friend is spending time on the phone or in location with a former

boy friend or even husband, he would see it as a red flag. And it is , because

some of us who with former girl friends can testify about how easy it is to

sleep with your former girl friend even if she is now married or with another

person. If am the man I would definitely run if my girl friend is talking with some one she calls or I know as a former mate. So most men with experience will believe that the union is perhaps dead immediately they see their girl friend with a former boy friend.   Any lady who don't want a sudden heartbreak must avoid this problem at all cost.

I remember a story a few years ago that happened to one of my friends in a pacific nation. There was a lady he befriended for some time and they had mutually broken up, and that was because the girl had met this other guy that was in the university and my friend was just an out door worker. But this guy and my friend lived in the same area and they do spoke to each other and this guy also knew that my friend dated the girl before.

Now the girl was coming to visit the university guy for the first time, and I guess the guy must have prepared well. Then this girl in order to prevent chaos, then told my friend that she was coming to visit her new boy friend and my friend told her he would also make sure she is totally welcomed. It should be noted that this lady never visited that area when she was dating my frend, they met at other places or her place and her excuse was the long distance, but here now she was coming there to visit the new guy. My friend had no problem because he believed the girl was above his pay grade. Then my friend when coming back home on that very day the girl called him to inform him of her visit in the coming days….., my friend said he thought he should check on university guy and joke about it and congratulate him, he branched and university guy met him and they dicuss and then my friend mentioned that Crystal (the girl) told him that she was visiting their area and that he is very happy for the university guy, and he told him to take care of her because she is a good girl. The university guy (if he was shocked, didn't show) greeted my friend and was just laughing about the whole issue and they left.

Then the girl arrived the following two day interval, she dressed beyond word and since my friend's place is the first on the street, she branched and greeted him and my friend told hershe should say hello to university guy. The girl Crystal left for her new guy place. But shockenly she met the doors locked and she checked around and when she tried to get him on cell phone, his phone was switched off. This lady became a bit stranded and very angry…….where is Thompson, she asked the people there and a woman told her that Thompson returned back to his school today and that it seems a bit too early as he don't return at that month. Crystal now dejected ran back to my friend and my friend was as shocked and he had the other number of Thompson, so he dialled him and Thompson picked up, my friend now told him whats on ground, but Thompson told my friend that he wasn't dating the girl and don't have any thing to do with her. He now asked my friend if the girl was in my friend's house and my friend said yes, and the university guy now asked why my friend was calling about a girl that came to visit him?. The girl later left distraught and frustrated. After three weeks of which the girl have ruminated and feel humiliated, she got through to him and she tried to cool her anger and spoke in soft tones on why he didn't tell he was going back to school. The university guy branded her a slut, that has unfinished business with her former boy friend, he quickly told her he has terminated and he was no longer interested! The girl pleaded with cries that she wont do that mistake again, but Thompson said he is not even angry at her, that his only pained was that he was stupid enough to think he can date another guy's girl friend. He said its over and cut her off. The lady cried for a long time and the guy went on to get another girl and this girl just roamed, and my friend noticed she just didn't come close to him that much, she never came to the area again.

So any lady who wants to mix up guys will probably lose all of them in one fell swope

The problem of financial impotency on the part of men is such that, the man may even leave the lady or end the relationship majorly because he can't bear to see her suffer under him! Many of my friends had this problem and it is a greate problem, in the sense that in most cases the man will not even tell the woman that the purpose am leaving you is because I can not cater for you with the resources that I have. The woman or some women having seen that the man is either jobless or under employed may still feel that the relationship can florish and there is no need to doubt or panic. But while the world is awashed with weak men who have lost that ancient instinct of men providing for their women and are prepared to live with her in audacious poverty and penury, some few men will not want that and will just feel some one else will be in a better position to provide for the lady.

But the catalyst factor that is at the top of quickly killing a man's interest in a romance is constant demand especially money!

With the present national and world inflation, most men are jobless or the data shows that women even have more job opportunities than men now and that statistically more women are in better jobs than men. What all these point to is the paucity of financially stable men that can take care of a family.

Thus ,it's obvious that ladies or women as a whole in this modern times must strive to be financially independent to cope with the growing problem of the jobless man.

This , I mean financial dependence of a lady on a man can also kill it. If a man is having financial challenge and he has a beautiful lady, he will start having pressure to take care of her, but if the lady her self is not patient and and turns into nagging, then the man may decide to end it or find another lady that will not be that problematic. This also happened with one of the ladies I had to end. I really like the lady but it came to a period where I was facing some financial problems and I was trying to find my way out and the lady became like a distraction and a cross that I could not continue. And she was never considerate of the situation and when I stop the relationship, she was heartbroken but I went incommunicado, and left the place.

Most men during the intro stage usually display temporal financial power, but most times this is a façade just to get the lady and I have friends who usually prepare written budgets when they want to get a particular lady, they will have a check book or logbook to calculate how much they intend to spend to get the job done and how much they have spent on it. So don't intend to spend that much after the did is done.

If a woman is totally depending on a man to meet her basic needs the she may be liable to heartbreak. Most men find it special to get a woman using money but that will hold if he finance remain constant ,the love remains hot and she marries her. But it becomes a problem if his finances drops drastically , the love dissipates due to any reason , she continues to demand recklessly or demands money for extravagance wastes or she is not married to him or have kids for him. Financial problem is one of the inevitable problems that strain any relationship and needs to be a center of focus

DISTANCE AND PROXIMITY

Now just as a close relationship can collapse due to romance fatigue, due to regular copulation or other routine, a relationship can also break down due to long distance or a wide distance location between the two parties. By this I mean if for instance, the man is living in another distance state or even country then the relationship may die gradually if they don't find a quick solution like relocation. Like if the woman left the man to work else where then the man may think of having a side chick to engage time and the side

chick may take things up a nutch and damage his previous relationship. And

on the other hand the lady may not be able to reject all the suitors who come

in the absence her boy friend.

Again the biggest problem with the long distance is that the trust and can

vanish as suspicion and jealousy take over. There are no easy ways to control

stability in a long distance relationship, you will just never know if your other

halve is faithful to you. And in most cases one or two of the two will do some

thing stupid. What I have seen really confirm this and it made me shiver.

A few years ago when I was doing my student housmanship, I left my city to

do it in another state. My father connected me to one of his former co worker

in a brewery industry. This man when i knew him was a married man with

kids, he was at that time what I knew was that , very devoted to church and

his wife and i never knew his wife then.

I met the man and he gave me a place to stay for the duration of my service

years. To cut it short , the man was staying in a pent house with like four

rooms with two other friends. They were co workers of a

telecommunications company and that was the company house. I was given the spare room to use. Then i noticed that when the go out for their jobs, they all came back in the night with hoes and street girls. I was shocked! Because even this my family friend was the most notorious among them, as he usually bring in two or three ladies for the night bang. When we spoke about his family, his wife, he made me understand that he don't joke with his wife and kids. He stated that he only saw his wife three times a year, when he goes to spend a week at home. So I understood he picked these unsafe girls to cover for his wife absence. Well, I took it well as there were so many preety ladies in that city and ofcourse the other men introduced me into the activity too. In times when I travel to visit home, this our family man will send me to his family and that was when I met his wife, however I must confess that his wife was not beautiful like that much and she lost some teeth! But I noticed how she also didn't show any concern about her husband absence, and infact I had to wait for her as she was out. I felt, well this man's home is as settled as he wanted and I counted him very lucky. I thought may be due to his wife's lack of overt beauty that's why his home front is peaceful. Again because the other men do have theirwives visit them from time to time, but he didn't do that and those onse always criticise him for that. They said he has abandoned his wife , but he told them, his wife wasn't complaining and that she understood he was here working his head off for the family. What I wanna bring out is this.......after I concluded my mission and returned home, I later heard the news from another unrelated family friend about how another man (also my father's friend) was now voraciously sleeping with our man's wife!

I was always aware of the moral kettle of this particular man but I never knew he could do such a thing as sleep with a married woman much less the wife of his friend, because they were both friends of my father.

This our man didn't know about this initially but, he later got wind that his so called gentle wife was being eaten daily by his former friend and this is when his powerlessness showed as both this man sleeping with his wife and his wife all accused him of sleeping with hundereds of girls himself in his work city. Our man had to run every where begging for help to salvage his family. I don't know whats happening now in that issue.

But if both parties are deeply connected, long distance will never be an issue. But , just as long distance is a recipe for disaster, a closer proximity cam also spell doom. But for the purpose of this topic, am not sure I want to write further on short distance , as this is usually a minor problem compared to long distance.

There are situations and they are the most fatal for relationships, that is when the parents of the man don't want the girl. If that is the case then on 7 over 10 that man will likely leave that girl. This happened to my. I had this lady I was so infatuated with and we have been having this thing for just nearly over seven months and my parents never knew about her, but they see her in church but , not with me and I was usually discret about it. Then as we got more into our selves , I was no longer discret , as i connected with her publicly in the church and then my mother saw this , she felt surprised and i don't even think it was an issue until we were at home. Then my mother told me that the lady was too wise for me , that she might be a slut. At first i didn't like her speaking negatively about my beautiful girl frend. But i did put her words to heart especially the slut thing because the girl was very beautiful. However the girl was very cool with me and never disturb my life, I mean she was just what I thought I needed in a girl. I didn't have much money then and the girl wasn't working but I just see that she wasn't nagging or showing any distress for my poverty . Then I want to go see her I use to call her on phone and tell her , and even though I had a routine of going to her place on Thursday I made sure I called her and whenever I got there I would meet her inside and I had to call her this way because her place of residence was very far from mine, I boarded like two cars to get there and she said she do go out some times. But i must say that I usually have this curousity , because her place was located deep inside a slum, the place was full of red eye touts, but I felt since she just arrived there to stay with her elder sister plus she don't speak the local dialet, that she wont be able to relate with these mess up people and she said the same thing as she laugh at their dirty and unhygienic life styles there.

Then I decided to pay her a visit on that same Thursday I usually go, but I have told her previously that I wasn't sure yet if I will come but that I will call her surely if I wanna come there and that was the routine. But I just said let me go and she knows the day.   But when I arrived I quietly got to her house and the place was locked and i thought I should waite a little, then I thought I should call her because I need to return on time to beat the traffic. I didn't have credit and I made to go and purchase, so as I was looking around, I saw this lady at meters away walking hand in hand comin toward her house, I quickly hid somewhere and watch till she came near and walk past with the tout towards her house !I stood up watch her go way down till she branched

with the man . I just went to the street and found a car and I returned home.

That's is how the relationship ended but upon her pleas, I didn't tell her that I

came, but I just told her am no longer interested.

Hence if friends show their hatred for a lady based on race or money or

status, then it would bear heavily on the mind of the man. But if the love is so

tight, then such issues will not derail. Infact most times love thrives from out

side aparthy. You can look at read about prince Harry of England who

renounced palace titles because they rejected his wife.

AGE DIFFERENCE

This one is one factor that quickly derails a relationship. For some men, they

may have a particular age in mind, for the type of lady they wanna move with.

But now love don't usually show on the face you know? So if they see a lady

they like, they may not be thinking about the age and their flustered brains

will be doing guess work and blanket their mind from connecting what they

see with their analytic faculty. What happen is that they may now be saddled

with a fake age in their mind. But let me say that if the woman is wise enough, she must not reveal her true age to the man, if her age is probably beyond the scale. In the mind some times age colours every thing and we must be very careful, that we don't destroy every thing by age. Age is a number, but again you must understand this fact......that every human has two running age.   The biological age and the natural age.

The biological age is the actual age or recorded age from birth and the natural age is the age of the person based on his trait makeup and nature's gift to them. We know that some people look far younger than their counterparts of the same age. Some people have a longer life expectancy. Now when some one is goner live to 90 years, you noticed that at 70 years they are looking very healthy and fit. But if some one wont live that long, then even from 50 years , they would start battling age related illness.

What am saying is if a woman realise that her man is having the wrong age about her in mind , then she shouldn't bother telling him some thing different as there won't be no benefit and all would be lost for nothing.

Now finally, what can say the last but not the least things that can lead to heartbreak are things that may have no remedy. These are issues from natural causes that are beyond a woman's pay grade.

Old age is an inevitable depreciation of physical attributes of attractiveness. In some few cases the man could be active, while the woman is no longer capable or no longer interested in romance activities. To that end, the man may move on to find some one else and the two of them could agree to such resolution and remain friends.

Sickness could also hinder the lady from being useful to the man. So if a young lady is suffering from a debilitating illness or long term health challenge that severely limits her activeness, then the man could move on. The lady at that point might be looking for comfort from the man, but the reality is that she may not get it once the man realise that she would be impaired long term or even short term.

Also if by an event of accident, the lady loses her romantic abilities, the men usually bails (runs away). Like I remember a lady who was so so beautiful and her boy friend was always fawning around her. Then she had an accident and broke one of her leg that required she work with crutches for years, the boy friend eloped away with another lady, who also was her friend who knew her

relationship with the man.

The next is a contribution from Peggy Adams

SIGNALS AND **RED LIGHTS** OF HEART BREAK

By Peggy Adams

1. <u>**Secret Phone calls**</u>- When a man is having an affair with another

   woman, what the lady will see is regular hidden phone calls. Now these

   phone calls are called hidden because, in most cases the lady may never

   know about them. Some men will look for convenient locations to pick

   calls from a secret lover, like their place of work, office, in the car, in

   the hotels, in rest rooms, in eating joints like Bigmac and burga

   kings….just any location out of his residence . Some men will even do

   these calls in the home, but will time it to when the lady is asleep or

   unaware. Some will do it while in the toilet or bath rooms. The main

   point is that if the lady becomes aware and suspicious, she will likely

   begin to note these calls. But for the most part, the lady is not suppose to know as the man will be extremely discret about it that it may go on for years and things will happen and she may not even know. A lady who had this problem, didn't know that any time she goes to work , her boy friend will just bring his other girl friend home and this went on for three years and she was just saved by concerned collegues of the man who exposed him. In essence a woman must critically look out for secret phone calls any way she can.

2. **<u>Celibacy</u>**- Celibacy is the state of abstaining from sex or marriage. Now when a man sees or meets a new lady his has falling for, then if the love or infatuation is great, what you will see is that he will most likely become celibate at home. Sex with his old girl friend will become boring to him, and he won't be able to pretend by having sex with her. But in some cases where the man knows that the cost of suspicion will be seriously damaging, he would continue the sex but his mind will mostly not be there. Some men will probably be able to satistfy multiple girl friends and keep the relationship.   But the point is that a lady should watch out for this if she senses a change in her man's sexual libido to negative. Infact based on experience, men who are having an affair that will break them from the old girl friend, will first

show their divided focus by not being able to perform on the bed the way they have been doing before. But a point of note is that a reduced libido could also be from other factors too, so a woman would just need to look very closely. But if a woman notices this signal, then the next action is to start monitoring the man, either personally or hiring people to do that for her. This is the time to check his phone and socio media and also his phone calls.

3. **<u>Long absence</u>**- when a man is about to break a woman's heart at any pont in time, he will start going to the events or persons that suits his interests. He will leave home at the drop of the slightest excuses, he won't to sit around the old girl friend for too long. He would drop a lot of fake excuses just to leave home and go meet the new love. Every woman will always remember the attention and telepathy that developed, the first time she met her lover or the love of her life. The man would have been very close, she could feel his heart beat and all that, she would also remember that the man will always crave to see her always and even distance was not in any way a a problem. Stopping those romantic activities from the man also doesn't mean the love is gone, as the love can become a routine. But it is also a signal if it is

becoming like a sought of detachment which was never the case before.

If a man was always detached from the beginning, then it is no problem.

But if he was a craven and suddenly he becomes invisible, then theres

need for a quick monitoring and investigation. If a woman becomes

alert at this stage, she may find out if it's a break up or just behavioural

change.

4. **<u>Checking out new girls</u>**- A man who is trying to double date of leave

his girl friend, will obviously start checking out new ladies, that's if he

hadn't done that in secret yet. This behaviour is a signal and very easy

to detect if the woman is alert. Now if a man has shown some of the

other signals, then the lady should watch out for the checking signal.

Even when he is with her, the man will unconsciously be checking

every girl passing. If they are both in the car, she will notice him double

checking every passing thing in skirt and the lady should spring into

monitoring mode to prevent unwanted actions.

5. **<u>Physical and emotional withdrawal</u>**- This is another clear signal that

London bridge is falling down. Infact, when the woman notices that

the man is no longer concern about how she feels, doesn't seem

interested in her tales, prefers to talk about the wind, then the woman should prepare to get her bags. The reason,i say pack the bags is based on my experience on this particular signal. When a man shows this kind of unfocused focus, then it may not be that he is looking to dump the woman in the immediate period, but what it could mean is that , he may already have another lady and may be he wish to keep the two or in most cases ,it could be that the present lady could be too much of an asset to discard, may be she is paying some of his bills , or may be she has a baby for him. He is not ready to drop her yet, but he will… eventually when her utility is over. So it s better to be the one to break his heart now rather than wait for the inevitable.

6. **<u>No longer pick calls</u>**- When the man is seriously seeing another girl, then he won't be interested in the calls of the present woman. He would still give snake oil excuses when confronted, but this kind of signal should be clear to any lady. However in most cases ladies don't get this signal until the did is done, they always blame it on the cell network or on the phone, or blame busy schedule. Agreed it may be nothing, but I always thread on the side of caution, especially if he never did that early in the relationship. Ofcourse , I know most men react to a lady's negative attitude on most cases. But but we are talking

on women holding the short stick, obviously many women are similarly problematic, but that is not what we looking at here. We are looking at women who are are doing their best to keep a man and not reciprocated.

7. **Limited or no physical presence**- At this stage , the man doesn't try to hid the fact that he don't want to be there with the lady, but as usual he may still concut several lame excuses why he ain't there, but it is left for the lady to see beyond the lies and run before the wolves arrives. The woman would just notice, she has not sat with her man in months and yet he is around her, or comes visiting. When a man loves a woman, he can do any thing to be close to her, just so if he now find her wortless, he will also do his best to steer clear of her. It is a very clear signal to any right thinking lady. Also if the lady tries to meet him up, he will throw up all sought of excuses and skip all chance of meeting, in fact he may start running away from her and she may not know. Some men are that bad.

8. **The new girl emerges**- If the lady continues to play dumb, and misses all those previous signals, then finally the second woman will come out of the shadows to claim what belongs to her, either subtly or overtly! It

may be the time to fight that lost battle or even burning the house down or even **kill Bill**.. A woman should not let this happen. Always better if she don't wait until the secret lady emerges otherwise the heartbreak is always more painful, since mostly the new woman may be totally not up to her level. Remember Prince Charles?

9. <u>**He says it is over**</u>- After the new woman emerges, it becomes rather how not when he will break the bad news to her that it is over. Some men may break it in different funny ways. We have seen some who told the old lady not to leave but to stay and form a three couple with the incoming lady, some thing that might be unacceptable. Any way he will tell her on phone or face to face that ok, you can find another man, am going this way.   Thanks for reading

1.SEEK FOR INNER LOVE NOT OUTWARD- A sensible lady who don't want to fall into the deep end of unwarranted heartbreak, it all starts from the kind of man you seeking for. Many ladies are carried away by lies and outward show. Some focus on those who infatuate about them without any deep love. It is hard to find such men but they exist and only needs a lady being very mobile. In essence a lady is adviced to exhibit the highest rate of awareness,so she can spot a man with a kindred spirit. Its not enough to be foolishly salivating for a bearded man, when infact a clean face man is the one salivating on you. Ladies that focus their attention on those little shining things don't ever get it right. You have to leave you greed for the sculptured man at the door and let your eyes meet a man who also likes you. There is always a man some where looking for you, yes we know that some ladies will rather focus on men who are not focusing on them with the idiotic hope that they will be able to capture such men to love them later. Such men don't last, or if you wanna keep such men, then you must be on your toes 24/7.

2.**KEEPING YOUR SELF OPEN TO NEW MEN**- some women believe in having only one man and that. A woman should be ready to keep are heart open to meeting the prince, despite having a man already. A better man is always on the way and you never know. A lady should not totally tye her self to a man not married to her. She has to keep her options open and that way she can easily move on if the present man begins to gaming.

3.**FIND OUT THE PROBLEMS THE MAN HAS** —A lady should try to know what problems the man has, these problems can lead to a break up and a lady should never be careless and believing that a man has no problem. Most of these troubled men have several inordinate addictions, some take drugs, some are addicted to gambling, some are porn addict, some are addicted to alcohol and some are suffering from inner ailements. Some are mentally challenged. You have to watchout because when a man has ailement or is addicted to drugs, cigar, gambling and alcohol, then there may be need to ask him to seek help or you may have to break up with him because such men are a basket of problem.

4.TRY TO KNOW HIS FAMILY- A lady that wanna survive need to try to guage the temperature of the family and how they see her. If the family look at her with contempt, then such relationship may hit the rock. Also the way the man defends the woman among the family, will also show his standing in the family and his interest in the relationship. If for instance , he has no influence at home in his family then that relationship could be very dangerious.

5. **MEET HIS FAMILY QUICKLY**-Another way to prevent unwanted variables is to priortise meeting the family of the man at any quickest opportunity, failure to do so quickly means you end upn playing second fiddle.

6.TRY TO DECIPHER WHAT HE LIKES MOST- Every man has his own point of interest and a lady should watch out to know what he seems to like and when he knows that you know what he likes and you are doing it often, he would also be more committed.

7.ALWAYS WORK TO LOOK MORE BEAUTIFUL- Every lady has that element of beauty, so its important that a lady check her self and those areas where a lady can make improvements, then she must continue to make improvements.   Most times that self improvement shows the man that the lady has not reach the level of diminishing returns yet. If a lady for any reason bordering on sheer carelessness, allows her self to become an old looking doddering hag, then she should not complain if the man starts the search for a new wine. A lady must instead see her self like a phoenix, which despite centuries of existence still mystifies the world by its splendour.

8. TRY TO WATCH HIS SPORT INTEREST- If possible a lady must develop interest in the particular sport of interest to then man. If the man loves soccer then the lady must study that sport and see if she can have interest there too, because if she loves it then the man will see another reason not to toy with her. Normally when a lady watches a sport with her man, it can take their love to a visceral level and keep both of them attached to each other.

9. **SAVE MONEY**-A lady must finally, be saving money, because you never know and if a break up happens then, there must be a part out of it. A lady should not lavish all her money in the name of love.

Now if a lady does all these things, it is expected that no man will ever take her for granted, but if by any means that man still chose to leave her then we will check out how to survive at our last issue.

1.**START A BUSINESS IF NO JOB**- A lady that has just lost a man ,must not sit idle and think about the loss. She needs to move on to some thing more profitable and it would restore her sanity. Get or focus on getting another job or start a new business and that way your mind will be unto some thing new, some thing more profitable. Also this can lead you to meet new set of people and keep your self wort.

2.**REMOVE AND DELETE ALL HIS THINGS**- A lady , at this stage should not be keeping any belongings of a departed man. All his pictures should be put away some where far. I will not encourage burning and if that is to be done to bring healing, then some few things can be speared for posterity. But just throw them away somewhere. If on social media, then the lady should block and remove him from her profile, delete his number totally and just close down every social media connection. When this is done, then you will be able to move on with your life, easily without the ghost of a man holding you down.

3. **LISTEN TO CLASSICAL MUSIC**- The lady who needs to occupy her mind can find instrumental classics to heal her heart. Music is a known healing substance and is very useful at this stage, especially instrumentals.

4. **A BETTER MAN AWAITING**- The truth is that in life, you will never see the very best people till death probably. I mean what ever good people you think you have seen, there are millions better out there and you just need to be ready to meet knew people and you will see that the man that wanted to destroy you was not even the sweetest thing that happened to you. There's always some one also searching for a woman like you. The assertion that "One man's Meat is another man's poison" is always an eternal truth. Those qualities of yours that probably made the previous man to quit could literally be what the next coming man is searching for, so there is no need to lose

heart over a man . In essence,every man is dispensible or even expendible, no man is an angel that you can not live without, especially the ones who don't seem to appreciate what ever you do.

5. **<u>GO CLUBBING</u>**-Its that time that a woman needs to enjoy her life, so clean up your self and dress to kill and go out to watch cinema, go to churches or mosque, go to orphanages, go to any recreational center, go out and brighten and enjoy your life and you will be surprised at the numerous men searching for a woman like you. I mean you will meet an upgrade or even the best of the best or you can even meet your real soul mate. Go out and enjoy your life.

6. **<u>LEARN AND IMPROVE FROM YOUR FAULTS</u>**- What is the worth of a breakup, if no lesson is learn't. Definitely there are a lot of things you did wrong and you know, even those you have to check out fro this book. You have to come out of any breakup, with a better version of you that will not repeat the mistakes of the past. That way, you will have a better chance next time. Now I mention this due to the common cases where a woman continues to be divorced from men consecutively like the kadashians? You must not be such a loose cannon.

7.**<u>MAKE YOUR SELF HAPPY</u>**- Don't let the break up matter al all, do all the above things and happiness will radiate your life and you will become like a new wine just arriving to the party. And I am sure you will like how every thing turned out.

Thanks every one, I have come to the conclusion of this book.

Contributors: Paul Hickman ,Peggy Adams

For enquiries:

Mail to leriorxewin@gmail.com